GASTRIC BYPASS COOKBOOK

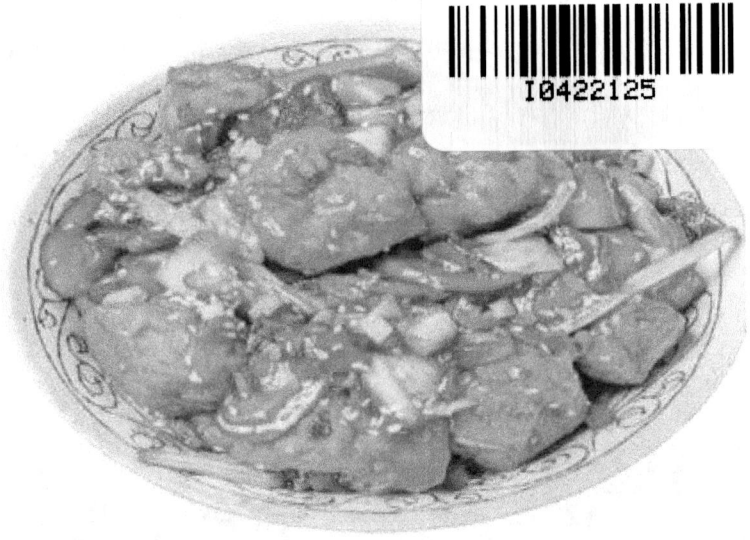

2000 Days Of Easy And Delicious
Recipes For All Ages To Prevent
Weight Gain After Bariatric Bypass
Surgery

Katherine J. Filer

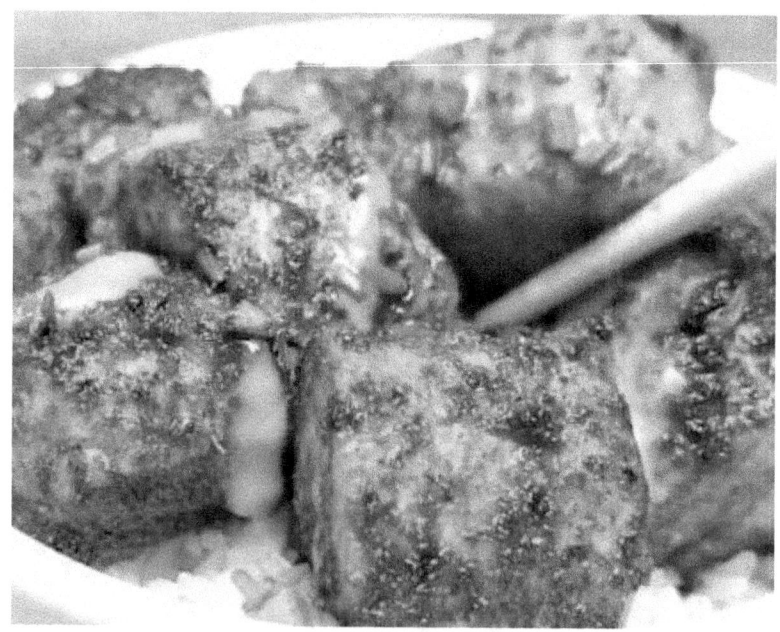

Table of Contents

INTRODUCTION

Embarking on a transformative journey towards health and vitality, envision a world where delicious, nourishing meals not only fuel your body but become the cornerstone of your post-gastric bypass success story. Picture this: savoring a delectable bite of a perfectly crafted dish that not only delights your taste buds but aligns seamlessly with the unique dietary needs of your revitalized self. Welcome to the Gastric Bypass Cookbook, a culinary compass designed to navigate the intricate landscape of post-surgery nutrition and make each meal a celebration of wellness.

Imagine the joy of discovering that your post-gastric bypass diet isn't about deprivation but about unlocking a world of flavorful possibilities that support your weight loss goals and overall health. In this cookbook, we delve into a symphony of ingredients and recipes meticulously curated to make your culinary experience both satisfying and nourishing. It's a guide that transcends the mundane, transforming your relationship with food into a journey of empowerment, vitality, and endless culinary creativity.

As we embark on this gastronomic adventure together, let's unlock the secrets to a post-gastric bypass lifestyle that's not just sustainable but truly enjoyable. From protein-packed wonders to nutrient-rich delights, each recipe is a testament to the idea that your culinary choices can be both beneficial and delicious. Say goodbye to monotony and hello to a world where vibrant flavors and optimal nutrition coexist harmoniously, guiding you towards a healthier, happier you.

The Gastric Bypass Cookbook is not merely a collection of recipes; it's a roadmap to a lifestyle where food becomes your ally in the pursuit of well-being. Get ready to embrace the kitchen with newfound excitement, as each page unfolds a culinary adventure designed to support your journey post-gastric bypass surgery. Let the joy of cooking and the magic of transformative flavors be your companions on this exciting path to a healthier, more vibrant you.

CHAPTER 1

Understanding Gastric Bypass

Gastric bypass is a surgical procedure designed to assist individuals in achieving significant and sustained weight loss by altering the digestive system. During the surgery, a small pouch is created at the top of the stomach, limiting its capacity and thus restricting food intake. Additionally, a section of the small intestine is rerouted to the new stomach pouch, affecting nutrient absorption. This procedure not only reduces the amount of food an individual can consume but also alters the digestive process, leading to physiological changes that contribute to weight loss.

The primary mechanism of gastric bypass involves two essential components: restriction and malabsorption. Restriction is achieved by creating a smaller stomach pouch, limiting the volume of food that can be comfortably consumed. This induces a feeling of fullness with smaller meals, promoting reduced calorie intake. Malabsorption results from the rerouting of the small intestine, decreasing the absorption of calories and nutrients. The bypassed portion of the intestine is responsible for absorbing a significant portion of nutrients from ingested food.

Understanding gastric bypass involves recognizing its potential benefits and challenges. While the procedure is highly effective in promoting weight loss and resolving obesity-related health issues, it requires a lifelong commitment to dietary and lifestyle changes. Adhering to a specific postoperative diet, characterized by smaller, nutrient-dense meals, is crucial to avoid complications such as nutrient deficiencies, dumping syndrome, and gastrointestinal discomfort.

Close collaboration with healthcare professionals, including dietitians and surgeons, is essential for individuals undergoing gastric bypass. Regular check-ups, nutritional monitoring, and ongoing support are integral components of a successful postoperative journey. By comprehending the intricate interplay of restriction and malabsorption, individuals can navigate the changes brought about by gastric bypass surgery, fostering not just weight loss but also improved overall health and well-being.

Foods To Eat And Avoid

Foods to Include:

1. Protein-Rich Foods:
- Protein is essential for maintaining muscle mass and promoting healing after surgery. Incorporate lean protein sources like poultry, fish, lean meats, eggs, and plant-based proteins such as beans and tofu. Aim for at least 60 to 80 grams of protein per day to meet nutritional requirements.

2. Non-Starchy Vegetables:
- Vegetables are rich in vitamins, minerals, and fiber while being low in calories. Opt for a variety of colorful, non-starchy vegetables like leafy greens, broccoli, cauliflower, and bell peppers. These foods contribute to overall health and help in preventing nutrient deficiencies.

3. Whole Grains:
- Choose whole grains over refined grains for sustained energy and better nutritional content. Quinoa, brown rice, oats, and whole wheat products provide essential nutrients, including fiber, which aids in digestion and helps maintain a healthy weight.

4. Low-Fat Dairy or Dairy Alternatives:
- Calcium is crucial for bone health, and individuals who have undergone gastric bypass surgery may be at risk for deficiencies. Include low-fat dairy products or fortified dairy

alternatives to meet calcium needs without excessive calories.

5. Healthy Fats:
- Incorporate sources of healthy fats such as avocados, nuts, seeds, and olive oil. These fats are essential for nutrient absorption and support overall well-being. However, moderation is key, as they are calorie-dense.

6. Hydration:
- Staying well-hydrated is vital, especially after gastric bypass surgery. Consume water regularly throughout the day to prevent dehydration and support the body's various functions. Adequate hydration aids in digestion, helps prevent constipation, and ensures overall well-being.

Foods to Avoid:

1. Highly Processed Foods:
- Processed foods often contain high levels of added sugars, unhealthy fats, and empty calories. Avoiding these can help control calorie intake and promote weight loss. Choose whole, nutrient-dense foods instead.

2. Sugary Foods and Beverages:
- High-sugar foods and drinks can lead to rapid spikes in blood sugar levels and contribute to unwanted weight gain. Steering clear of sugary items like candies, pastries, and

sweetened beverages is crucial for managing postoperative health.

3. Carbonated Beverages:
- Carbonated drinks can cause discomfort and may lead to stretching of the stomach pouch post-surgery. Opt for still water and other non-carbonated, non-caloric beverages to stay hydrated without risking digestive issues.

4. High-Fat and Fried Foods:
- Foods high in unhealthy fats and deep-fried items can be challenging to digest and contribute to weight regain. Limit intake of fried foods, processed snacks, and fatty cuts of meat to support weight loss and overall health.

5. Large Meals:
- Eating large meals can strain the stomach pouch and lead to discomfort. Opt for smaller, more frequent meals to ensure proper nutrient absorption and avoid overstretching the digestive system.

Core Benefits Of Following A Gastric Bypass Cookbook

1. Effective Weight Loss:
- One of the primary goals of gastric bypass surgery is significant and sustained weight loss. The prescribed diet helps control caloric intake, promoting weight loss and the reduction of obesity-related health risks.

2. Nutrient Absorption Optimization:
- Gastric bypass surgery alters the digestive tract, impacting the absorption of nutrients. Following the prescribed diet ensures that individuals receive essential vitamins and minerals, preventing nutrient deficiencies and supporting overall health.

3. Prevention of Dumping Syndrome:
- Dumping syndrome is a common side effect of gastric bypass surgery, characterized by rapid emptying of stomach contents into the small intestine. Adhering to the recommended diet helps prevent dumping syndrome, minimizing symptoms like nausea, sweating, and diarrhea.

4. Balanced Macronutrient Intake:
- The diet emphasizes a balanced intake of macronutrients, particularly protein. Adequate protein is essential for

maintaining muscle mass, supporting healing, and preventing the loss of lean body mass during weight loss.

5. Prevention of Complications:
- Following a gastric bypass diet helps prevent complications associated with the surgery, such as malnutrition, anemia, and vitamin deficiencies. Proper nutrition supports the healing process and reduces the risk of postoperative complications.

6. Stable Blood Sugar Levels:
- The diet encourages the consumption of low-glycemic foods, which helps stabilize blood sugar levels. This is particularly important for individuals with diabetes or those at risk of developing diabetes after surgery.

7. Improved Digestive Tolerance:
- Adhering to a gastric bypass diet involves gradually introducing and testing various foods to determine individual tolerances. This approach helps identify foods that may cause discomfort or digestive issues, allowing for a more personalized and well-tolerated diet.

8. Promotion of Lifestyle Changes:
- The diet serves as a foundation for long-term lifestyle changes, promoting healthier eating habits and portion control. Establishing these habits early on contributes to sustained weight management and overall well-being.

9. Enhanced Quality of Life:

- Successful adherence to a gastric bypass diet contributes to improved physical health, increased energy levels, and enhanced overall quality of life. Weight loss and the resolution of obesity-related conditions can lead to improved mobility and a more active lifestyle.

10. Professional Guidance and Support:

- Following a gastric bypass diet involves ongoing support from healthcare professionals, including dietitians and nutritionists. Regular check-ins and monitoring help individuals make informed choices, ensuring they stay on track with their dietary goals.

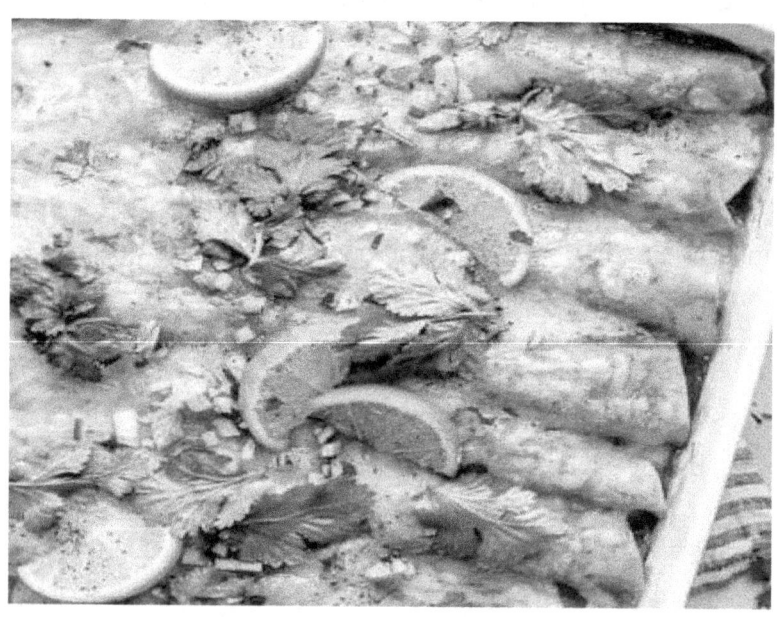

20 Healthy Shopping Ingredients For A Gastric Bypass Diet

1. Lean Proteins:
- Chicken Breast: High in protein, low in fat.
- Turkey: Lean source of protein.
- Fish (Salmon, Cod, and Tuna): Rich in omega-3 fatty acids.
- Lean Ground Beef or Turkey: Protein without excess fat.

2. Low-Fat Dairy or Dairy Alternatives:
- Greek Yogurt: High in protein.
- Skim Milk or Almond Milk: Calcium without added fats.
- Low-Fat Cheese: A source of calcium and protein.

3. Whole Grains:
- Quinoa: High in protein and fiber.
- Brown Rice: Rich in fiber and nutrients.
- Oats: Complex carbohydrates for sustained energy.

4. Vegetables:
- Leafy Greens (Spinach, Kale): Packed with vitamins and minerals.
- Broccoli: High in fiber and antioxidants.
- Bell Peppers: Colorful and rich in vitamin C.

5. Fruits:

- Berries (Blueberries, Strawberries): Low in sugar, high in antioxidants.
- Apples: High in fiber and vitamins.
- Kiwi: Vitamin C-rich and easy to digest.

6. Healthy Fats:
- Avocado: Provides healthy fats and nutrients.
- Olive Oil: A source of monounsaturated fats.

7. Nuts and Seeds:
- Almonds: Healthy fats and protein.
- Chia Seeds: Omega-3 fatty acids and fiber.

8. Protein Supplements:
- Whey Protein Powder: Supports protein intake.
- Plant-Based Protein Powder: Suitable for vegetarian options.

9. Eggs:
- Egg Whites: High-quality protein, low in fat.

10. Canned or Dry Legumes:
- Black Beans, Chickpeas: Excellent sources of plant-based protein.

11. Sugar-Free or Low-Sugar Items:
- Stevia or Monk Fruit Sweetener: For sweetening without added sugars.

12. Hydration Options:
- Water: Essential for hydration.
- Herbal Tea: A low-calorie beverage option.

13. Herbs and Spices:
- Cilantro, Basil, Rosemary: Add flavor without extra calories.

14. Low-Sodium Broths:
- Chicken or Vegetable Broth: Useful for cooking and hydration.

15. Non-Starchy Vegetables:
- Zucchini, Cauliflower, Asparagus: Low in calories, high in nutrients.

16. Tomato Products:
- Canned Diced Tomatoes: A versatile ingredient with various uses.

17. Sugar-Free Sauces:
- Sugar-Free Ketchup, Mustard, Hot Sauce: Flavor without added sugars.

18. Seafood:
- Shrimp, Cod, Tuna: Low in fat, high in protein.

19. Cottage Cheese:

- Low-Fat Cottage Cheese: A good source of protein and calcium.

20. Ground Flaxseed:
- Flaxseed: Provides omega-3 fatty acids and fiber.

Complications Of Gastric Bypass If The Right Diet Isn't Adopted

1. Nutrient Deficiencies:
- Inadequate nutrient intake due to poor dietary choices can lead to deficiencies in essential vitamins and minerals. Common deficiencies include iron, vitamin B12, calcium, and vitamin D, which can result in anemia, osteoporosis, and other health issues.

2. Dumping Syndrome:
- Dumping syndrome occurs when food, especially sugar-rich or high-fat items, moves too quickly from the stomach to the small intestine. Symptoms include nausea, vomiting, diarrhea, and abdominal cramps. Avoiding certain foods and eating smaller, well-balanced meals can help prevent dumping syndrome.

3. Dehydration:
- Reduced stomach size and changes in the digestive system may limit the body's ability to absorb water. Failure

to stay adequately hydrated can lead to dehydration, impacting overall health and potentially causing complications such as kidney stones.

4. Malnutrition:
- Poor dietary choices or insufficient nutrient intake can result in malnutrition. Malnutrition can have serious consequences, affecting energy levels, immune function, and overall well-being. Regular monitoring of nutritional status and adherence to dietary guidelines are crucial for preventing malnutrition.

5. Gastrointestinal Issues:
- The altered anatomy post-gastric bypass surgery can make certain foods challenging to tolerate. Consuming foods that are too fibrous, high in fats, or difficult to digest may cause gastrointestinal discomfort, bloating, and other digestive issues.

6. Weight Regain:
- Without proper adherence to a healthy diet, individuals may experience weight regain. This can occur when high-calorie, low-nutrient foods are consumed in excess, negating the benefits of the surgery and impacting long-term weight management.

7. Stomach Pouch Stretching:

- Overeating or consuming large quantities of food can lead to stretching of the stomach pouch created during surgery. This can compromise the effectiveness of the procedure and contribute to weight regain.

8. Psychological Impact:

- Failing to follow the recommended diet may lead to emotional and psychological challenges. Feelings of guilt, frustration, or disappointment can arise, impacting mental health and potentially contributing to disordered eating patterns.

9. Reflux and Gastritis:

- Consuming acidic or irritating foods may lead to reflux or gastritis. These conditions can cause discomfort, inflammation, and potentially damage the esophagus or stomach lining.

10. Increased Risk of Complications:

- Poor dietary habits can increase the risk of postoperative complications, including infections, healing issues, and prolonged recovery times.

CHAPTER 2

30 DAYS MEAL PLAN

Week 1:
- Day 1:
  - Breakfast: Protein-Packed Omelette
  - Lunch: Grilled Chicken Salad
  - Dinner: Baked Lemon Herb Chicken

- Day 2:
  - Breakfast: Chia Seed Pudding
  - Lunch: Quinoa and Vegetable Stir-Fry
  - Dinner: Vegetable and Tofu Stir-Fry

- Day 3:
  - Breakfast: Cottage Cheese and Pineapple Bowl
  - Lunch: Salmon and Asparagus Foil Pack
  - Dinner: Salmon and Quinoa Bowl

- Day 4:
  - Breakfast: Quinoa Breakfast Bowl
  - Lunch: Turkey Lettuce Wraps
  - Dinner: Zucchini Noodles with Turkey Bolognese

- Day 5:
  - Breakfast: Turkey and Veggie Scramble
  - Lunch: Vegetarian Quinoa Bowl
  - Dinner: Mushroom and Spinach Stuffed Chicken Breast

- Day 6:
  - Breakfast: Smoothie Bowl
  - Lunch: Egg Salad Lettuce Wraps
  - Dinner: Cauliflower Crust Veggie Pizza

- Day 7:
  - Breakfast: Egg Muffins
  - Lunch: Mushroom and Spinach Quiche Cups
  - Dinner: Shrimp and Broccoli Quinoa Bowl

Week 2:

- Day 8:
  - Breakfast: Spinach and Feta Breakfast Wrap
  - Lunch: Quinoa and Vegetable Stir-Fry
  - Dinner: Vegetable and Tofu Stir-Fry

- Day 9:
  - Breakfast: Chia Seed Pudding
  - Lunch: Turkey Lettuce Wraps
  - Dinner: Zucchini Noodles with Turkey Bolognese

- Day 10:
- Breakfast: Sweet Potato Hash
- Lunch: Egg Salad Lettuce Wraps
- Dinner: Mushroom and Spinach Stuffed Chicken Breast

- Day 11:
- Breakfast: Mexican Breakfast Casserole
- Lunch: Vegetarian Quinoa Bowl
- Dinner: Cauliflower Crust Veggie Pizza

- Day 12:
- Breakfast: Smoothie Bowl
- Lunch: Mushroom and Spinach Quiche Cups
- Dinner: Shrimp and Broccoli Quinoa Bowl

- Day 13:
- Breakfast: Egg Muffins
- Lunch: Grilled Chicken Salad
- Dinner: Baked Lemon Herb Chicken

- Day 14:
- Breakfast: Avocado and Smoked Salmon Toast
- Lunch: Turkey and Cheese Roll-Ups
- Dinner: Turkey and Sweet Potato Skillet

Week 3:

- Day 15:
  - Breakfast: Quinoa Breakfast Bowl
  - Lunch: Salmon and Asparagus Foil Pack
  - Dinner: Salmon and Quinoa Bowl

- Day 16:
  - Breakfast: Turkey and Veggie Scramble
  - Lunch: Egg Salad Lettuce Wraps
  - Dinner: Zucchini Noodles with Turkey Bolognese

- Day 17:
  - Breakfast: Smoothie Bowl
  - Lunch: Grilled Chicken Salad
  - Dinner: Baked Lemon Herb Chicken

- Day 18:
  - Breakfast: Egg Muffins
  - Lunch: Vegetarian Quinoa Bowl
  - Dinner: Mushroom and Spinach Stuffed Chicken Breast

- Day 19:
  - Breakfast: Sweet Potato Hash
  - Lunch: Quinoa and Vegetable Stir-Fry
  - Dinner: Cauliflower Crust Veggie Pizza

- Day 20:
  - Breakfast: Mexican Breakfast Casserole
  - Lunch: Turkey Lettuce Wraps
  - Dinner: Shrimp and Broccoli Quinoa Bowl

- Day 21:
  - Breakfast: Cottage Cheese and Pineapple Bowl
  - Lunch: Mushroom and Spinach Quiche Cups
  - Dinner: Turkey and Sweet Potato Skillet

Week 4:

- Day 22:
  - Breakfast: Avocado and Smoked Salmon Toast
  - Lunch: Turkey and Cheese Roll-Ups
  - Dinner: Cauliflower Crust Veggie Pizza

- Day 23:
  - Breakfast: Greek Yogurt Parfait with Berries
  - Lunch: Mushroom and Spinach Quiche Cups
  - Dinner: Shrimp and Broccoli Quinoa Bowl

- Day 24:
  - Breakfast: Quinoa Breakfast Bowl
  - Lunch: Grilled Chicken Salad
  - Dinner: Baked Lemon Herb Chicken

- Day 25:
  - Breakfast: Chia Seed Pudding
  - Lunch: Vegetarian Quinoa Bowl

- Dinner: Mushroom and Spinach Stuffed Chicken Breast

- Day 26:
  - Breakfast: Smoothie Bowl
  - Lunch: Turkey Lettuce Wraps
  - Dinner: Zucchini Noodles with Turkey Bolognese

- Day 27:
  - Breakfast: Egg Muffins
  - Lunch: Salmon and Asparagus Foil Pack
  - Dinner: Salmon and Quinoa Bowl

- Day 28:
  - Breakfast: Cottage Cheese and Pineapple Bowl
  - Lunch: Quinoa and Vegetable Stir-Fry
  - Dinner: Turkey and Sweet Potato Skillet

- Day 29:
  - Breakfast: Greek Yogurt Parfait with Berries
  - Lunch: Turkey Lettuce Wraps
  - Dinner: Mushroom and Spinach Stuffed Chicken Breast

Day 30:
  - Breakfast: Chia Seed Pudding with Mango
  - Lunch: Grilled Chicken Salad
  - Dinner: Baked Lemon Herb Chicken

CHAPTER 3

BREAKFAST RECIPES

Protein-Packed Omelette

- Ingredients:

- 2 large eggs
- 1/4 cup diced turkey or chicken breast
- 1/4 cup chopped spinach
- 1 tablespoon feta cheese

- Preparation:

- Whisk eggs and pour into a non-stick pan.
- Add diced turkey, spinach, and feta.
- Cook until eggs are set.

- Nutritional Value: High protein, low carbs.

Cooking Time: 10 minutes.

Spinach and Feta Breakfast Wrap

- Ingredients:

- 1 whole wheat tortilla
- 2 eggs, scrambled
- 1/4 cup sautéed spinach
- 1 tablespoon crumbled feta

- Preparation:

- Fill tortilla with scrambled eggs, spinach, and feta.
- Roll into a wrap.

- Nutritional Value: Balanced protein and carbs.

Cooking Time: 7 minutes.

Chia Seed Pudding

- Ingredients:

- 2 tablespoons chia seeds
- 1/2 cup almond milk
- 1/4 teaspoon vanilla extract
- 1/4 cup sliced strawberries

- Preparation:

- Mix chia seeds, almond milk, and vanilla.
- Refrigerate overnight.
- Top with sliced strawberries before serving.

- **Nutritional Value:** High in omega-3, low carbs.

Prep Time: 5 minutes.

Cottage Cheese and Pineapple Bowl

- Ingredients:

- 1/2 cup low-fat cottage cheese
- 1/2 cup diced pineapple
- 1 tablespoon chopped nuts (almonds or walnuts)

- Preparation:

- Combine cottage cheese, pineapple, and nuts.
- Mix well and serve.

- Nutritional Value: High protein, low carbs.

Prep Time: 3 minutes.

Quinoa Breakfast Bowl

- Ingredients:

- 1/2 cup cooked quinoa
- 1/4 cup almond milk
- 1 tablespoon chia seeds
- 1/4 cup diced mango

- Preparation:

- Mix cooked quinoa with almond milk and chia seeds.
- Top with diced mango.

- Nutritional Value: Protein and fiber-rich, low carbs.

Prep Time: 7 minutes.

Turkey and Veggie Scramble

- Ingredients:

- 2 large eggs
- 1/4 cup ground turkey
- 1/4 cup diced bell peppers
- 1/4 cup diced tomatoes

- Preparation:

- Scramble eggs in a pan, add ground turkey, bell peppers, and tomatoes.
- Cook until eggs are fully cooked.

- Nutritional Value: High protein, low carbs.

Cooking Time: 8 minutes.

Smoothie Bowl

- Ingredients:

- 1/2 cup unsweetened almond milk
- 1/2 frozen banana
- 1/4 cup berries (blueberries, raspberries)
- 1 tablespoon almond butter

- Preparation:

- Blend almond milk, frozen banana, berries, and almond butter.
- Pour into a bowl and add toppings if desired.

- Nutritional Value: Protein, healthy fats, and antioxidants.

Prep Time: 5 minutes.

Egg Muffins

- **Ingredients:**
  - 3 eggs
  - 1/4 cup diced ham
  - 1/4 cup chopped spinach
  - 1/4 cup shredded cheddar cheese

- **Preparation:**

  - Whisk eggs and mix with ham, spinach, and cheese.
  - Pour into muffin tin and bake until set.

- **Nutritional Value:** High protein, low carbs.

Cooking Time: 15 minutes.

Avocado and Smoked Salmon Toast

- Ingredients:

- 1 slice whole grain bread
- 1/4 ripe avocado, mashed
- 2 slices smoked salmon
- 1 teaspoon capers

- Preparation:

- Toast bread and spread mashed avocado on top.
- Add smoked salmon and sprinkle with capers.

- Nutritional Value: Healthy fats, omega-3, and protein.

Prep Time: 5 minutes.

Sweet Potato Hash

- Ingredients:

- 1/2 cup sweet potato, grated
- 2 eggs
- 1/4 cup diced bell peppers
- 1 tablespoon olive oil

- Preparation:

- Sauté grated sweet potato and bell peppers in olive oil until tender.
- Create wells in the hash and crack eggs into them.
- Cook until eggs are done to your liking.

- **Nutritional Value:** Complex carbs, protein, and healthy fats.

Cooking Time: 15 minutes.

Mexican Breakfast Casserole

- Ingredients:

- 2 eggs, beaten
- 1/4 cup black beans, drained and rinsed
- 1/4 cup diced tomatoes
- 1 tablespoon chopped cilantro

- Preparation:

- Mix beaten eggs with black beans, diced tomatoes, and cilantro.
- Bake in a dish until eggs are set.

- Nutritional Value: Protein, fiber, and fresh flavors.

Cooking Time: 20 minutes.

LUNCH RECIPES

Grilled Chicken Salad

- Ingredients:

- 4 oz grilled chicken breast, sliced
- 2 cups mixed salad greens
- 1/4 cup cherry tomatoes, halved
- 1/4 cup cucumber, sliced
- 1 tablespoon balsamic vinaigrette

- Preparation:

- Grill chicken and slice it.
- Toss salad greens, cherry tomatoes, and cucumber.
- Top with grilled chicken and drizzle with vinaigrette.

- Nutritional Value: High protein, low carbs.

Prep Time: 15 minutes.

Quinoa and Vegetable Stir-Fry

- Ingredients:

- 1/2 cup cooked quinoa
- 1/4 cup broccoli florets
- 1/4 cup bell peppers, sliced
- 1/4 cup snap peas
- 2 tablespoons low-sodium soy sauce

- Preparation:

- Stir-fry vegetables in a pan until slightly tender.
- Add cooked quinoa and soy sauce, stir until well combined.

- Nutritional Value: Balanced protein and carbs.

Cooking Time: 10 minutes.

Salmon and Asparagus Foil Pack

- Ingredients:

- 4 oz salmon fillet
- 1/2 cup asparagus spears
- 1 tablespoon olive oil
- Lemon slices, salt, and pepper to taste

- Preparation:

- Place salmon and asparagus on a foil sheet.
- Drizzle with olive oil, add lemon, salt, and pepper.
- Seal the foil and bake until salmon is cooked.

- Nutritional Value: Omega-3 fatty acids, high protein.

Cooking Time: 20 minutes.

Turkey Lettuce Wraps

- Ingredients:

- 4 oz ground turkey
- 1/4 cup diced bell peppers
- 1/4 cup shredded carrots
- Lettuce leaves for wrapping
- 1 tablespoon hoisin sauce

- Preparation:

- Cook ground turkey with bell peppers and carrots.
- Spoon the mixture into lettuce leaves.
- Drizzle with hoisin sauce before serving.

- Nutritional Value: Lean protein, low carbs.

Cooking Time: 12 minutes.

Vegetarian Quinoa Bowl

- Ingredients:

- 1/2 cup cooked quinoa
- 1/4 cup black beans, drained and rinsed
- 1/4 cup corn kernels
- 1/4 cup cherry tomatoes, halved
- 2 tablespoons cilantro, chopped

- Preparation:

- Combine quinoa, black beans, corn, tomatoes, and cilantro.
- Mix well and serve.

- **Nutritional Value:** Plant-based protein, fiber, and antioxidants.

Prep Time: 10 minutes.

Egg Salad Lettuce Wraps

- Ingredients:

- 2 hard-boiled eggs, chopped
- 1/4 cup celery, finely diced
- 1 tablespoon Greek yogurt
- Lettuce leaves for wrapping

- Preparation:

- Mix chopped eggs, celery, and Greek yogurt.
- Spoon into lettuce leaves for a low-carb wrap.

- Nutritional Value: Protein-rich, low carbs.

Prep Time: 10 minutes.

Mushroom and Spinach Quiche Cups

- **Ingredients:**

  - 3 eggs
  - 1/4 cup almond milk
  - 1/4 cup mushrooms, chopped
  - 1/4 cup spinach, chopped

- **Preparation:**

  - Whisk eggs with almond milk, then mix in mushrooms and spinach.
  - Pour into muffin tin and bake until set.

- **Nutritional Value:** Protein-packed, low carbs.

Cooking Time: 20 minutes.

Shrimp and Avocado Salad

- Ingredients:

- 4 oz grilled shrimp
- 1/2 avocado, sliced
- 2 cups mixed greens
- 1 tablespoon olive oil

- Preparation:

- Grill shrimp until cooked.
- Toss mixed greens with sliced avocado and grilled shrimp.
- Drizzle with olive oil before serving.

- Nutritional Value: Healthy fats, high protein.

Prep Time: 15 minutes.

Cauliflower Fried Rice with Chicken

- Ingredients:

- 1 cup cauliflower rice
- 4 oz cooked chicken, diced
- 1/4 cup peas and carrots, mixed
- 2 tablespoons soy sauce

- Preparation:

- Sauté cauliflower rice, chicken, peas, and carrots in a pan.
- Add soy sauce and stir until heated through.

- Nutritional Value: Low carbs, moderate protein.

Cooking Time: 12 minutes.

Tuna and Cucumber Rolls

- Ingredients:

- 1 can tuna, drained
- 1/4 cup Greek yogurt
- 1 cucumber, sliced lengthwise
- 1 tablespoon chopped dill

- Preparation:

- Mix tuna with Greek yogurt and dill.
- Spoon onto cucumber slices and roll.

- Nutritional Value: Protein-rich, low carbs.

Prep Time: 10 minutes.

DINNER RECIPES

Baked Lemon Herb Chicken

- Ingredients:

  - 6 oz. chicken breast
  - 1 tablespoon olive oil
  - 1 teaspoon dried thyme
  - 1 teaspoon dried rosemary
  - Juice of 1 lemon

- **Preparation:**

  - Marinate chicken with olive oil, thyme, rosemary, and lemon juice.
  - Bake in the oven until chicken is cooked through.

- **Nutritional Value:** Lean protein, healthy fats.

Cooking Time: 25 minutes.

Vegetable and Tofu Stir-Fry

- Ingredients:

- 1/2 cup firm tofu, cubed
- 1 cup broccoli florets
- 1/2 cup bell peppers, sliced
- 1/4 cup low-sodium soy sauce

- Preparation:

- Stir-fry tofu, broccoli, and bell peppers in a pan.
- Add soy sauce and cook until vegetables are tender.

- Nutritional Value: Plant-based protein, low carbs.

Cooking Time: 15 minutes.

Salmon and Quinoa Bowl

- Ingredients:

- 4 oz salmon fillet
- 1/2 cup cooked quinoa
- 1/4 cup cherry tomatoes, halved
- 1/4 cup cucumber, diced

- Preparation:

- Grill or bake salmon until cooked.
- Assemble a bowl with quinoa, cherry tomatoes, and cucumber.
- Top with cooked salmon.

- **Nutritional Value:** Omega-3 fatty acids, protein.

Cooking Time: 20 minutes.

Zucchini Noodles with Turkey Bolognese

- **Ingredients:**

  - 1 cup zucchini noodles
  - 4 oz ground turkey
  - 1/2 cup tomato sauce (no added sugar)
  - 1/4 teaspoon dried oregano

- **Preparation:**

  - Cook ground turkey in a pan until browned.
  - Add tomato sauce and oregano, simmer until heated through.
  - Serve over zucchini noodles.

- **Nutritional Value:** Lean protein, low carbs.

Cooking Time: 15 minutes.

Mushroom and Spinach Stuffed Chicken Breast

- Ingredients:

- 2 chicken breasts
- 1/2 cup mushrooms, chopped
- 1 cup spinach, wilted
- 1/4 cup feta cheese

- Preparation:

- Butterfly chicken breasts and stuff with mushrooms, spinach, and feta.
- Bake until chicken is cooked through.

- Nutritional Value: Protein, vegetables, and calcium.

Cooking Time: 30 minutes.

Cauliflower Crust Veggie Pizza

- Ingredients:

- 1 cup cauliflower rice
- 1/4 cup mozzarella cheese
- 1/4 cup tomato sauce (no added sugar)
- 1/4 cup bell peppers, sliced

- Preparation:

- Mix cauliflower rice with cheese to form a crust.
- Top with tomato sauce and sliced bell peppers.
- Bake until crust is crispy and cheese is melted.

- Nutritional Value: Low carbs, vegetables.

Cooking Time: 25 minutes.

Shrimp and Broccoli Quinoa Bowl

- **Ingredients:**

  - 1/2 cup cooked quinoa
  - 4 oz. shrimp, peeled and deveined
  - 1 cup broccoli florets
  - 1 tablespoon olive oil

- **Preparation:**

  - Sauté shrimp and broccoli in olive oil until cooked.
  - Serve over a bed of cooked quinoa.

- **Nutritional Value:** Protein, fiber, and healthy fats.

Cooking Time: 15 minutes.

Turkey and Sweet Potato Skillet

- Ingredients:

- 4 oz. ground turkey
- 1/2 cup sweet potato, diced
- 1/4 cup black beans, drained and rinsed
- 1/4 teaspoon cumin

- Preparation:

- Cook ground turkey in a skillet, add sweet potato and black beans.
- Season with cumin and cook until sweet potatoes are tender.

- Nutritional Value: Lean protein, complex carbs.

Cooking Time: 20 minutes.

Eggplant and Chickpea Curry

- Ingredients:

- 1 cup eggplant, diced
- 1/2 cup chickpeas, drained and rinsed
- 1/4 cup coconut milk
- 1 tablespoon curry powder

- Preparation:

- Sauté eggplant and chickpeas, then add coconut milk and curry powder.
- Simmer until eggplant is cooked through.

- Nutritional Value: Plant-based protein, fiber.

Cooking Time: 25 minutes.

Stuffed Bell Peppers with Turkey

- Ingredients:

- 2 bell peppers, halved
- 4 oz. ground turkey
- 1/2 cup quinoa, cooked
- 1/4 cup salsa (no added sugar)

- Preparation:

- Cook ground turkey, mix with cooked quinoa and salsa.
- Stuff bell peppers with the mixture and bake until peppers are tender.

- **Nutritional Value:** Lean protein, whole grains, vegetables.

Cooking Time: 30 minutes.

DESSERTS AND TREATS RECIPES

Greek Yogurt Parfait with Berries

- Ingredients:

- 1/2 cup Greek yogurt
- 1/4 cup mixed berries (blueberries, strawberries)
- 1 tablespoon chopped nuts (almonds or walnuts)

- Preparation:

- Layer Greek yogurt with mixed berries in a glass.
- Top with chopped nuts.

- **Nutritional Value:** Protein-rich, antioxidants.

Prep Time: 5 minutes.

Avocado Chocolate Mousse

- Ingredients:

- 1 ripe avocado
- 2 tablespoons unsweetened cocoa powder
- 2 tablespoons honey or agave nectar

- Preparation:

- Blend avocado, cocoa powder, and honey until smooth.
- Chill in the refrigerator before serving.

- Nutritional Value: Healthy fats, antioxidants.

Prep Time: 10 minutes.

Baked Cinnamon Apple Slices

- Ingredients:

- 1 apple, thinly sliced
- 1/2 teaspoon cinnamon
- 1 teaspoon honey

- Preparation:

- Toss apple slices with cinnamon and honey.
- Bake until apples are soft.

- Nutritional Value: Fiber, natural sweetness.

Cooking Time: 15 minutes.

Chia Seed Pudding with Mango

- Ingredients:

- 2 tablespoons chia seeds
- 1/2 cup almond milk
- 1/4 teaspoon vanilla extract
- 1/4 cup diced mango

- Preparation:

- Mix chia seeds, almond milk, and vanilla. Refrigerate overnight.
- Top with diced mango before serving.

- **Nutritional Value:** Omega-3, fiber, and natural sweetness.

Prep Time: 5 minutes.

Protein-Rich Peanut Butter Balls

- Ingredients:

- 1/2 cup peanut butter
- 1/4 cup protein powder
- 2 tablespoons honey
- 1/4 cup crushed nuts (almonds or peanuts)

- Preparation:

- Mix peanut butter, protein powder, and honey until well combined.
- Form into small balls and roll in crushed nuts.

- Nutritional Value: Protein, healthy fats.

Prep Time: 15 minutes.

Coconut Chia Seed Popsicles

- Ingredients:

- 2 tablespoons chia seeds
- 1 cup coconut milk
- 1 tablespoon shredded coconut
- 1 tablespoon agave syrup

- Preparation:

- Mix chia seeds, coconut milk, shredded coconut, and agave syrup.
- Pour into popsicle molds and freeze until solid.

- Nutritional Value: Omega-3, fiber, and tropical flavor.

Prep Time: 5 minutes.

Almond Flour Banana Bread

- Ingredients:

- 1 cup almond flour
- 2 ripe bananas, mashed
- 2 eggs
- 1/4 cup unsweetened almond milk

- Preparation:

- Mix almond flour, mashed bananas, eggs, and almond milk.
- Bake in a loaf pan until a toothpick comes out clean.

- Nutritional Value: Gluten-free, protein, and natural sweetness.

Cooking Time: 30 minutes.

Berry Yogurt Ice Cream

- Ingredients:

- 1 cup mixed berries (strawberries, blueberries, raspberries)
- 1 cup Greek yogurt
- 1 tablespoon honey

- Preparation:

- Blend mixed berries, Greek yogurt, and honey.
- Freeze the mixture in an ice cream maker or a shallow dish, stirring occasionally.

- Nutritional Value: Protein, antioxidants.

Prep Time: 10 minutes.

Pumpkin Spice Energy Bites

- Ingredients:

- 1/2 cup canned pumpkin puree
- 1/4 cup almond flour
- 1/4 cup oats
- 1 tablespoon pumpkin spice

- Preparation:

- Mix pumpkin puree, almond flour, oats, and pumpkin spice.
- Form into small balls and refrigerate until firm.

- Nutritional Value: Fiber, seasonal flavors.

Prep Time: 15 minutes.

Chocolate Avocado Pudding

- Ingredients:

- 2 ripe avocados
- 1/4 cup unsweetened cocoa powder
- 1/4 cup maple syrup
- 1 teaspoon vanilla extract

- Preparation:

- Blend avocados, cocoa powder, maple syrup, and vanilla until creamy.
- Chill in the refrigerator before serving.

- Nutritional Value: Healthy fats, antioxidants.

Prep Time: 10 minutes.

SNACKS RECIPES

Cheesy Cauliflower Bites

- Ingredients:

- 2 cups cauliflower florets
- 1/2 cup grated Parmesan cheese
- 1 teaspoon garlic powder
- 1/4 teaspoon black pepper

- Preparation:

- Toss cauliflower with Parmesan, garlic powder, and black pepper.
- Bake until cauliflower is golden and crispy.

- Nutritional Value: Low-carb, calcium.

Cooking Time: 20 minutes.

Protein-Packed Hummus

- **Ingredients:**

  - 1 can chickpeas, drained
  - 1/4 cup tahini
  - 1/4 cup olive oil
  - Juice of 1 lemon

- **Preparation:**

  - Blend chickpeas, tahini, olive oil, and lemon juice until smooth.
  - Serve with sliced veggies or whole-grain crackers.

- **Nutritional Value:** Protein, healthy fats.

Prep Time: 10 minutes.

Turkey and Cheese Roll-Ups

- Ingredients:

- 4 slices deli turkey
- 4 slices cheese (cheddar or Swiss)
- 1/4 cup baby spinach leaves

- Preparation:

- Lay turkey slices flat, add a slice of cheese and a few spinach leaves on each.
- Roll up and secure with toothpicks.

- Nutritional Value: Protein, calcium.

Prep Time: 5 minutes.

Crunchy Roasted Chickpeas

- Ingredients:

- 1 can chickpeas, drained and dried
- 1 tablespoon olive oil
- 1 teaspoon cumin
- 1/2 teaspoon smoked paprika

- Preparation:

- Toss chickpeas with olive oil, cumin, and smoked paprika.
- Roast until crispy, shaking the pan occasionally.

- Nutritional Value: Protein, fiber.

Cooking Time: 30 minutes.

Cucumber and Greek Yogurt Bites

- Ingredients:

- 1 cucumber, sliced
- 1/2 cup Greek yogurt
- 1 tablespoon fresh dill, chopped

- Preparation:

- Mix Greek yogurt with chopped dill.
- Top cucumber slices with the yogurt mixture.

- **Nutritional Value:** Protein, low-calorie.

Prep Time: 5 minutes.

Apple and Almond Butter Sandwiches

- Ingredients:

- 1 apple, sliced
- 2 tablespoons almond butter
- 1 tablespoon chia seeds

- Preparation:

- Spread almond butter on apple slices and create sandwiches.
- Sprinkle chia seeds on top for added texture.

- **Nutritional Value:** Fiber, healthy fats, and protein.

Prep Time: 5 minutes.

Caprese Skewers

- Ingredients:

- Cherry tomatoes
- Mozzarella cheese balls
- Fresh basil leaves
- Balsamic glaze for drizzling

- Preparation:

- Thread cherry tomatoes, mozzarella balls, and basil leaves onto skewers.
- Drizzle with balsamic glaze before serving.

- Nutritional Value: Calcium, antioxidants.

Prep Time: 10 minutes.

Edamame

- Ingredients:

- 1 cup edamame, steamed
- Sea salt to taste

- Preparation:

- Steam edamame until tender.
- Sprinkle with sea salt before enjoying.

- Nutritional Value: Protein, fiber.

Cooking Time: 5 minutes.

Berry and Cottage Cheese Parfait

- Ingredients:

- 1/2 cup low-fat cottage cheese
- 1/4 cup mixed berries (strawberries, blueberries)
- 1 tablespoon honey (optional)

- Preparation:

- Layer cottage cheese and mixed berries in a glass.
- Drizzle with honey if desired.

- Nutritional Value: Protein, antioxidants.

Prep Time: 5 minutes.

Seaweed Snack Rolls

- Ingredients:

- Roasted seaweed sheets
- 1/4 cup avocado, sliced
- 1/4 cup cucumber, julienned

- Preparation:

- Place avocado and cucumber on a seaweed sheet.
- Roll tightly and slice into bite-sized pieces.

- Nutritional Value: Omega-3, fiber.

Prep Time: 5 minutes.

BEVERAGES AND DRINKS RECIPES

Green Tea Citrus Cooler

- Ingredients:

- 1 green tea bag
- 1 cup hot water
- 1/4 cup orange juice
- Ice cubes

- Preparation:

- Steep the green tea bag in hot water and let it cool.
- Mix with orange juice and pour over ice.

- **Nutritional Value:** Antioxidants, vitamin C.

Prep Time: 5 minutes.

Cucumber Mint Infused Water

- Ingredients:

- 1/2 cucumber, sliced
- 1/4 cup fresh mint leaves
- 1.5 liters water
- Ice cubes

- Preparation:

- Combine cucumber slices and mint leaves with water.
- Refrigerate for a few hours before serving over ice.

- Nutritional Value: Hydration, refreshing.

Prep Time: 5 minutes (+ chilling time).

Protein-Packed Berry Smoothie

- Ingredients:

- 1/2 cup mixed berries (strawberries, blueberries)
- 1/2 cup Greek yogurt
- 1/2 cup almond milk
- 1 scoop protein powder

- Preparation:

- Blend berries, Greek yogurt, almond milk, and protein powder until smooth.
- Pour into a glass and enjoy.

- Nutritional Value: Protein, antioxidants.

Prep Time: 5 minutes.

Iced Peppermint Herbal Tea

- Ingredients:

- 1 peppermint tea bag
- 1 cup hot water
- 1/4 cup unsweetened almond milk
- Ice cubes

- Preparation:

- Steep the peppermint tea bag in hot water and let it cool.
- Add almond milk and pour over ice.

- Nutritional Value: Digestive aid, dairy-free.

Prep Time: 5 minutes.

Golden Turmeric Latte

- Ingredients:

- 1 cup unsweetened almond milk
- 1/2 teaspoon ground turmeric
- 1/4 teaspoon cinnamon
- 1/4 teaspoon ginger powder
- 1 teaspoon honey (optional)

- Preparation:

- Heat almond milk, turmeric, cinnamon, and ginger in a pan.
- Whisk until well combined, add honey if desired.

- Nutritional Value: Anti-inflammatory, dairy-free.

Prep Time: 7 minutes.

Berry-Lemon Detox Water

- Ingredients:

- 1/2 cup mixed berries (blueberries, raspberries)
- 1/2 lemon, sliced
- Fresh mint leaves
- 1.5 liters water
- Ice cubes

- Preparation:

- Combine berries, lemon slices, and mint leaves with water.
- Refrigerate for a few hours before serving over ice.

- Nutritional Value: Hydration, antioxidants.

Prep Time: 5 minutes (+ chilling time).

Vanilla Almond Protein Shake

- Ingredients:

- 1 cup unsweetened almond milk
- 1 scoop vanilla protein powder
- 1/4 teaspoon almond extract
- Ice cubes

- Preparation:

- Blend almond milk, protein powder, and almond extract until smooth.
- Pour into a glass over ice.

- Nutritional Value: Protein, low carbs.

Prep Time: 3 minutes.

Minty Green Detox Smoothie

- Ingredients:

- 1/2 cup cucumber, sliced
- 1/2 cup kale leaves
- 1/2 green apple, cored and sliced
- 1/2 lemon, juiced
- 1 cup water

- Preparation:

- Blend cucumber, kale, green apple, lemon juice, and water until smooth.
- Strain if desired and serve over ice.

- Nutritional Value: Hydration, antioxidants.

Prep Time: 5 minutes.

Iced Matcha Latte

- Ingredients:

- 1 teaspoon matcha powder
- 1 cup unsweetened almond milk
- 1/2 teaspoon honey (optional)
- Ice cubes

- Preparation:

- Whisk matcha powder with a little hot water until smooth.
- Add almond milk and honey, then pour over ice.

- Nutritional Value: Antioxidants, dairy-free.

Prep Time: 5 minutes.

Pineapple Ginger Sparkler

- Ingredients:

- 1/2 cup pineapple chunks
- 1/2 teaspoon freshly grated ginger
- Sparkling water
- Ice cubes

- Preparation:

- Muddle pineapple chunks and grated ginger in a glass.
- Top with sparkling water and ice.

- Nutritional Value: Refreshing, aids digestion.

Prep Time: 5 minutes.

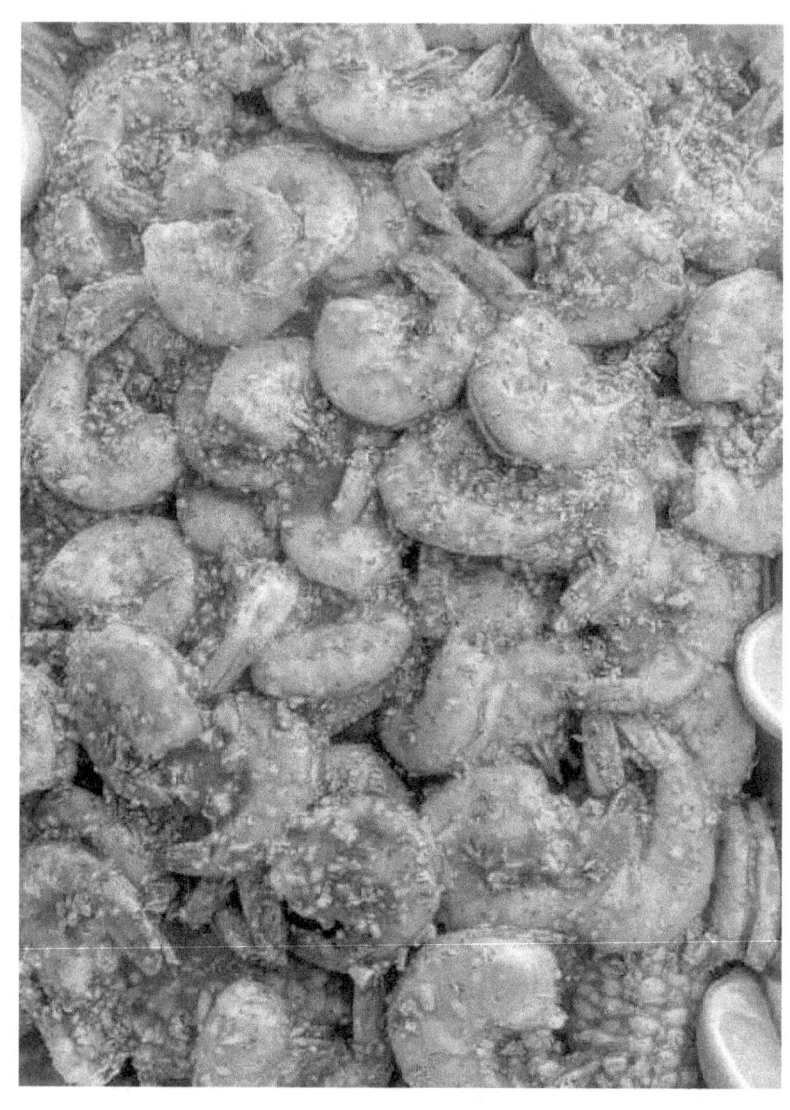

CONCLUSION

In conclusion, the journey towards health and well-being after undergoing gastric bypass surgery is undoubtedly transformative, and the recipes in this gastric bypass cookbook serve as a valuable companion on this path. With a focus on nutrient-dense ingredients, balanced flavors, and mindful portion sizes, these recipes are crafted to support post-surgery dietary needs while ensuring a diverse and enjoyable culinary experience.

This cookbook not only provides a diverse array of breakfasts, lunches, dinners, desserts, snacks, and beverages but also emphasizes the importance of nutritional value. From protein-packed meals to refreshing beverages, each recipe has been thoughtfully curated to align with the nutritional requirements post-gastric bypass surgery. The incorporation of lean proteins, healthy fats, and a variety of fruits and vegetables ensures a well-rounded approach to maintaining optimal health.

As you embark on this gastronomic journey, remember that each recipe is a testament to the commitment to a healthier lifestyle. The culinary adventures outlined in this cookbook aim not only to tantalize taste buds but also to inspire a sense of empowerment and ownership over one's well-being. Beyond the kitchen, these recipes are a celebration of resilience and the pursuit of a life filled with vitality and joy.

To our readers, may the pages of this cookbook be more than just a collection of recipes – may they be a source of motivation and a reminder that each dish prepared is a step towards a healthier and happier you. Embrace the flavors, savor the moments, and let this cookbook be a constant companion on your journey to a revitalized and nourished life. Your commitment to health is commendable, and with each recipe, you're not just cooking; you're crafting a future filled with wellness, one delicious meal at a time.

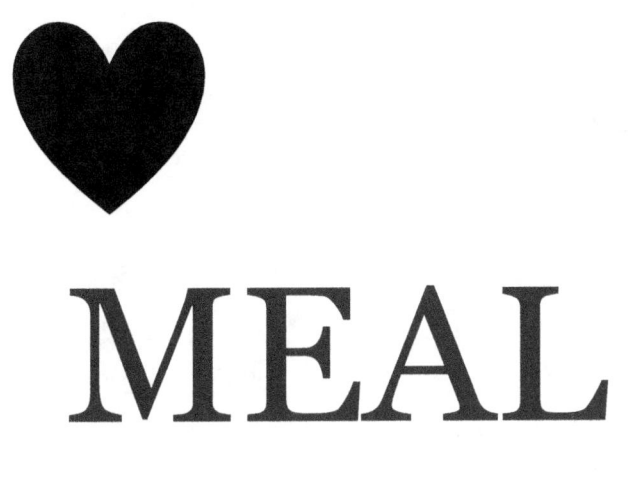

MEAL

TRACKER

	Breakfast	Lunch	Dinner
Monday			

	Breakfast	Lunch	Dinner
Tuesday			

	Breakfast	Lunch	Dinner
Wednesday			

	Breakfast	Lunch	Dinner
Thursday			

	Breakfast	Lunch	Dinner
Friday			

	Breakfast	Lunch	Dinner
Saturday			

	Breakfast	Lunch	Dinner
Sunday			

	Breakfast	Lunch	Dinner
Monday			

	Breakfast	Lunch	Dinner
Tuesday			

	Breakfast	Lunch	Dinner
Wednesday			

	Breakfast	Lunch	Dinner
Thursday			

	Breakfast	Lunch	Dinner
Friday			

	Breakfast	Lunch	Dinner
Saturday			

	Breakfast	Lunch	Dinner
Sunday			

	Breakfast	Lunch	Dinner
Monday			

	Breakfast	Lunch	Dinner
Tuesday			

	Breakfast	Lunch	Dinner
Wednesday			

	Breakfast	Lunch	Dinner
Thursday			

	Breakfast	Lunch	Dinner
Friday			

	Breakfast	Lunch	Dinner
Saturday			

	Breakfast	Lunch	Dinner
Sunday			

Monday	Breakfast	Lunch	Dinner

Tuesday	Breakfast	Lunch	Dinner

Wednesday	Breakfast	Lunch	Dinner

Thursday	Breakfast	Lunch	Dinner

Friday	Breakfast	Lunch	Dinner

Saturday	Breakfast	Lunch	Dinner

Sunday	Breakfast	Lunch	Dinner

	Breakfast	Lunch	Dinner
Monday			

	Breakfast	Lunch	Dinner
Tuesday			

	Breakfast	Lunch	Dinner
Wednesday			

	Breakfast	Lunch	Dinner
Thursday			

	Breakfast	Lunch	Dinner
Friday			

	Breakfast	Lunch	Dinner
Saturday			

	Breakfast	Lunch	Dinner
Sunday			

Monday	Breakfast	Lunch	Dinner

Tuesday	Breakfast	Lunch	Dinner

Wednesday	Breakfast	Lunch	Dinner

Thursday	Breakfast	Lunch	Dinner

Friday	Breakfast	Lunch	Dinner

Saturday	Breakfast	Lunch	Dinner

Sunday	Breakfast	Lunch	Dinner

	Breakfast	Lunch	Dinner
Monday			

	Breakfast	Lunch	Dinner
Tuesday			

	Breakfast	Lunch	Dinner
Wednesday			

	Breakfast	Lunch	Dinner
Thursday			

	Breakfast	Lunch	Dinner
Friday			

	Breakfast	Lunch	Dinner
Saturday			

	Breakfast	Lunch	Dinner
Sunday			

Monday	Breakfast	Lunch	Dinner

Tuesday	Breakfast	Lunch	Dinner

Wednesday	Breakfast	Lunch	Dinner

Thursday	Breakfast	Lunch	Dinner

Friday	Breakfast	Lunch	Dinner

Saturday	Breakfast	Lunch	Dinner

Sunday	Breakfast	Lunch	Dinner

	Breakfast	Lunch	Dinner
Monday			

	Breakfast	Lunch	Dinner
Tuesday			

	Breakfast	Lunch	Dinner
Wednesday			

	Breakfast	Lunch	Dinner
Thursday			

	Breakfast	Lunch	Dinner
Friday			

	Breakfast	Lunch	Dinner
Saturday			

	Breakfast	Lunch	Dinner
Sunday			

Monday	Breakfast	Lunch	Dinner

Tuesday	Breakfast	Lunch	Dinner

Wednesday	Breakfast	Lunch	Dinner

Thursday	Breakfast	Lunch	Dinner

Friday	Breakfast	Lunch	Dinner

Saturday	Breakfast	Lunch	Dinner

Sunday	Breakfast	Lunch	Dinner

www.ingramcontent.com/pod-product-compliance
Lightning Source LLC
Chambersburg PA
CBHW071209290526
45796CB00008B/194